Warm Up

The Key to Injury Free Exercise

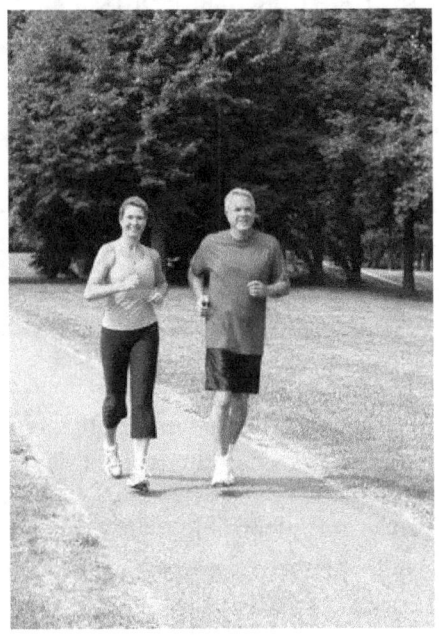

Health Learning Series

M. Usman

Mendon Cottage Books

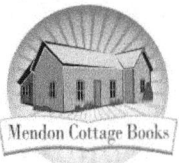

JD-Biz Publishing

Disclaimer

The information is this book is provided for informational purposes only. It is not intended to be used and medical advice or a substitute for proper medical treatment by a qualified health care provider. The information is believed to be accurate as presented based on research by the author.

The contents have not been evaluated by the U.S. Food and Drug Administration or any other Government or Health Organization and the contents in this book are not to be used to treat cure or prevent disease.

The author or publisher is not responsible for the use or safety of any diet, procedure, or treatment mentioned in this book. The author or publisher is not responsible for errors or omissions that may exist.

Warning

The Book is for informational purposes only and before taking on any diet, treatment, or medical procedure, it is recommended to consult with your primary health care provider.

Our books are available at
1. Amazon.com
2. Barnes and Noble
3. Itunes
4. Kobo
5. Smashwords
6. Google Play Books

Table of Contents

Preface

Performing warm ups before any high intensity physical activity, sports, or exercises, is important in a multitude of ways. A good, fulfilling session of warm up exercises will make sure that the body does not go into the energy-demanding phase of an exercise or workout too swiftly. There will be a gradual increase in your heart rate, which will steadily increase the flow of blood in your muscles, and other parts of the body, preparing you both physically and mentally for an injury free exercise. The importance of a workout can be compared simply to the analogy of a car being driven in cold weather; what people tend to do is, allow their cars to warm up before picking up high speeds. The same principle, in a slightly modified sense, applies to a workout. For a strenuous and demanding workout, its best to physically prepare yourself, by steadily increasing the body's temperature with patience.

By giving your body a nice warm up with many of the techniques like jogging, walking, etc., you are in fact improving blood circulation within different joints, muscles, and tendons, much like oiling a squeaky wheel. With the increased blood flow, the heart rate also rises and the muscles warm up to prevent any injury from taking place. Moreover, warm up exercises also have a psychological affect and they prepare your brain by easing it into the physical activities that are soon to follow. This is extremely helpful in exercises like weight lifting, high intensity running, and aerobics.

The body and mind thus synchronize and ease into the workout making sure that no part of the body faces any injury as a result of the exercises that are soon to follow. Keep reading on and find out the details of a warm up.

Getting Started

Chapter # 1: Benefits of Warming Up

Warming up, cooling down, and stretching are all essential but overlooked parts of a complete exercise, workout, or training program. Even though these components are not at all exhaustive, they in fact get a person ready for an injury free exercise. Most people skip over them and feel out of shape during the main exercise. These are often called forgotten techniques as most training centers are usually filled with people skipping to the main course instead of these.

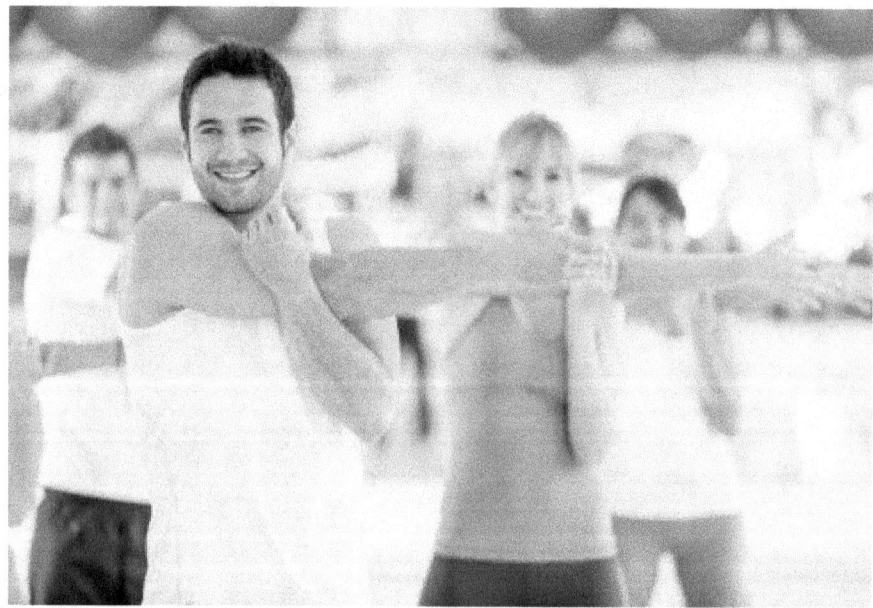

Warming up has many benefits; the main one is primarily focused on is injury prevention due to increased amount of blood flow in the muscles of the body. But, don't take a warm up as just a safety measure, as a well-done warm up is necessary to peak one's performance during the main course of the exercise. The benefits include:

✓ **Raised Muscle Temperature** – The muscles that are actively engaged during a warm up have a greater temperature giving them greater force during contracts and more ease during relaxations. In this way, both the muscle's strength and speed can be enhanced. Moreover, the chances of a muscle overstretching, resulting in an injury, are also reduced.

✓ **Dilation of Blood Vessels** – As the blood vessels dilate, the resistance to blood flow drops, along with decreased amounts of stress on the heart.

✓ **More Efficient Cooling** – Warming up kicks off the heat dissipation mechanisms in the body, which then allows an athlete's body to cool more efficiently. Thus, when a real even arises, the athlete can perform with greater dexterity and delay the time taken by the body to overheat.

✓ **Increased Blood Temperature** – The temperature of blood vessels also increases due to greater movement. The increase in blood temperature results in the bond between hemoglobin and oxygen to weaken, making oxygen more available to the working muscles.

✓ **Greater Range of Motion** – Range of motion is defined as the distance a person can achieve between the flexed positions of his/her joint to the extended position of the joint. For instance, during a bicep curl, the full range of a person's motion begins with an upright arm and ends with the weight coming down to the shoulder. The range of motion can be increased using warm up exercises that focus on flexibility to loosen up the chronically tight muscles.

✓ **Hormonal Changes** – For regulating the processes involved during energy production, the body increases the production of certain hormones. During warm up exercises, the hormones balance each other, making more fatty acids and carbohydrates available for energy production afterwards.

✓ **Mental Preparation** – A warm up not only physically enables the body to perform demanding tasks, but also enables it to increase its mental performance by clearing one's mind, reviewing skills, increasing focus, and maintaining strategy.

Chapter # 2: Stretching

So there's a warm up routine, then the main physical activity followed by a stretch routine? That's right. Stretches are even more over looked than warm ups, as they are considered something that only aerobic athletes can take advantage of. Almost all of the lifters want to jump right into their workouts and do not pay much needed attention to warm ups, or in some cases stretches, that follow. Stretching is necessary for the body, as it prevents a lot of problems that can develop over time due to increased physical activity like muscle soreness, tightness, and to body builders, the common problem known as "muscle bound".

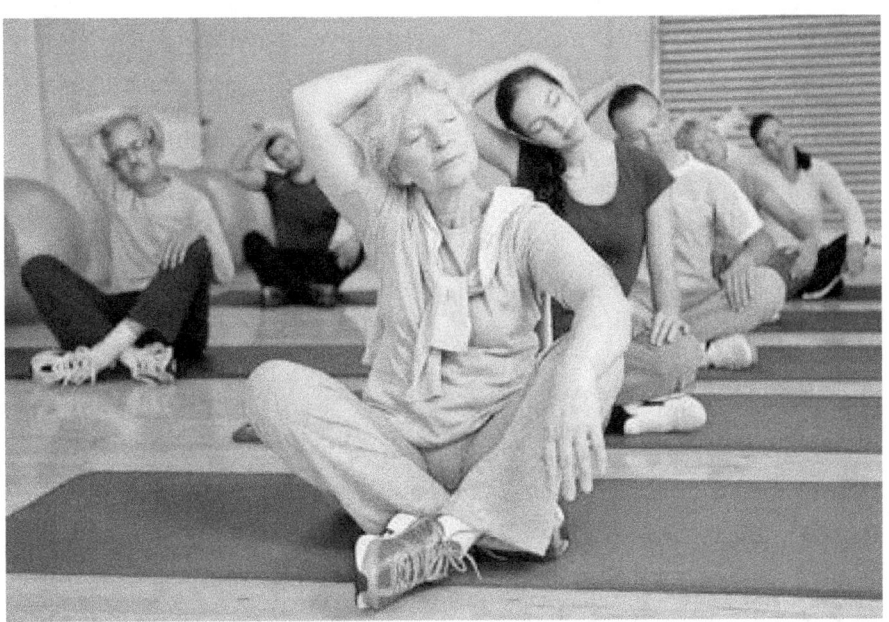

Stretches have the ability to loosen up a muscle that can become tight during a workout. This prevents injury to the muscle in the post-workout time period. It is a proven fact that stretching can decrease the amount of muscle soreness that follows a workout or physical activity. Not only has it been proven theoretically, but also athletes, like weight lifters, have testified to the fact. Thus, in order to effectively limit the amount of muscle soreness, a painful stretch is necessary, but in the long term, only you will gain. Decide for yourself; is it better to be gritting your teeth during a 30-second stretch after a workout, or to be gritting your teeth all day because of all the normal activities that now induce pain?

When bodybuilders workout, it is generally thought that they will lose their muscle flexibility and become "muscle bound". This is no myth and if a bodybuilder fails to stretch properly, he/she will fall victim to this trap. The trap itself might not be that harmful, but think for yourself; why lose flexibility when you can gain it with just a few minutes of extra work. Two of the greatest bodybuilders of all time, Tom Platz and Arnold Schwarzenegger, have relied heavily on stretching to get a fully developed and mobile muscle. Both the monster lifters based their routines on the fact that if a muscle can stretch more, it can contract more. In the words of Arnold Schwarzenegger, "Bodybuilders like Ed Corney, known as perhaps the best poser in modern bodybuilding, could never move with such beauty if their muscles, tendons, and ligaments were tight and constricted". Moreover, it has been proven time and again that muscle separation can be cured through stretching which extensively develops as time progresses. Thus, stretching is effective and necessary for all individuals indulged in any type of physical workout.

Post or Pre-workout stretching?

Nowadays, there is a lot of controversy surrounding pre-workout stretching. The truth of the matter is that a light stretch regiment will not adversely affect a person's physical performance. Before a workout, in order to achieve the best out of your muscles, focus on a light intensity stretch that won't push your muscles to the limits. If you do stretch too much in an initial, non-contracted position, you will only damage your performance in the real activity. Furthermore, before a workout, as there is not that much amount of blood flow in the muscles required for an optimum stretch, you will only damage your muscles in the endeavor.

It has been agreed from all sides that a stretch after a workout is best to increase the mobility of muscles. After a workout, the muscles can get greatly stiff and thus sore. Therefore, to prevent any long-term effects of this soreness, a post-workout stretch is necessary. The muscles are fully pumped with blood that gives them a better range of motion and reduces every negative impact of the exercise carried out before. As stretching of a muscle is simply caused by a pull due to an antagonist muscle, after the lengthening phase of an exercise, the muscles are fully stretched thus a post workout stretch should focus primarily on relaxing the muscle. The details of a complete stretching plan have been given in the next section.

Chapter # 3: Types of Stretches

There are many types of stretches, with each stretch having its own dedicated fan following. Many people swear to one type, while some to the others. The three basic stretches along with their merits and de-merits have been given below:

1.   **Ballistic Stretching:**

The name pretty much says it all. This type of stretching involves forcing a muscle way past its limit by using techniques like jerking and bouncing. This is a common sight when someone is lying down or standing up, trying to get a hold of his/her foot. The person literally presses his/her back to reach the required length, using momentum to get close to the destination. This is a quite dangerous version of stretching and should be avoided as much as possible. Some people, however, like to push their bodies to the limits, which is the primary reason why this type of stretching is chosen.

2.   **Static Stretching:**

Static stretching, on the other hand, is a much safer and controlled way of stretching. There is a very minimal chance of getting a muscle injury, and it is very beneficial if one plans on increasing his/her flexibility. Static stretching includes almost all muscle groups and the entire exercise lasts from 5 – 10 minutes. Static stretching is performed by placing the muscle under tension. The muscles in front of and behind the concerned muscles are first relaxed. They are then brought under tension, where they are held there for a few seconds to increase their length.

3.   **Dynamic Stretching:**

This form of stretching is highly effective, but has a lot of risk for injury, if executed incorrectly. However, these are not similar to the ballistic stretches, as these movements always involve the person being in control of the exercise and never crossing the pain threshold. Furthermore, dynamic stretches are kept dynamic as they are specific for each type of sport and particular for every activity. It's the final part of the warm up and its objective is to gain peak mental and physical performance.

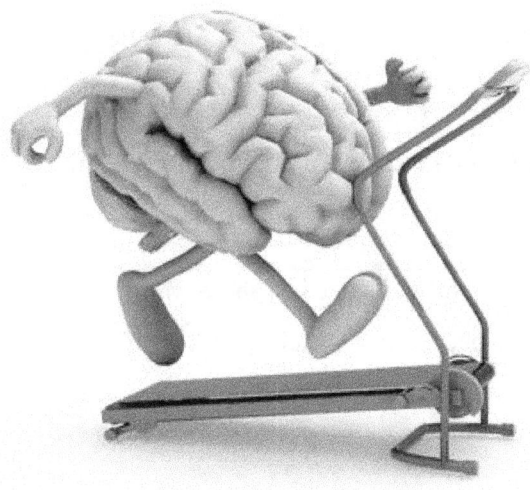

How to Warm Up

Chapter # 1: Intro

The forthcoming warm up exercises are thought out in an organized manner, to raise your body temperature along with the rate of breathing and blood pumping. The warm ups enable the body to wake-up and mobilize the joints, muscle fibers, and tendons for the physical activity that is soon to begin. The warm up is short and will not last more than 10 minutes, but it has benefits that last for the complete time period of the workout.

The 4 stages of the warm up are as follows:

1.   **Mobility Exercises** – these are the gentle movements that will be undertaken to give greater mobility to your joints.

2.   **Pulse Raising** – these are processes that will raise the heart rate through aerobic activity.

3.   **Targeted Mobility Exercise** – these warm ups focus on the muscle groups that need to be used during the main course of the exercise. These warm ups are more dynamic and focused than those in stage 1.

4.   **Final Pulse Raising** – this is the last stage of the warm up and will focus on increasing the heart rate along with the body temperature so that the body will be all geared up for the oncoming activity.

Chapter # 2: Mobility Exercises

This is the first stage of the warm up regimen and is performed while the person is stationary. The purpose of this particular warm up routine is to gently mobilize all the joints in the body. To reach ultimate efficiency, try to perform each movement 4 to 6 times with each limb, wherever relevant.

1. **Neck:**

    Stand tall and begin by dropping your head, first to the left side and then to the right, directly. Then, turn it to the left and then to the right followed by moving it backwards and then dropping your chin to the chest. Finally, rotate your head from left to right and then right to left.

2. **Shoulders:**

    Stand tall and begin by rolling your shoulders from the front to the back several times. Next, lift your shoulders up towards your ears, and then lower them. Repeat this a few times. Finally, rotate your shoulders back and down, making your chest stick out slightly. This is the correct position for good posture.

3. **Hips:**

    Stand with your legs a little wider than your hips and start to make a big circle with the help of your hips. Do this in both directions and then lift one knee up to the front, rotate this leg out to the side and then repeat this with the other leg. Place the leg down and repeat the hip swings.

4. **Trunk:**

Stand with the feet at hip width, bring your arms to the waist and rotate the torso the right and then to the left. Repeat this 5 – 6 times while making sure that the hips remain at a central position. Next, drop your hands first to the sides and try to reach as down as possible with your hand while making sure that the hands remain in contact with your thighs. Bend your trunk towards each side alternately, again making sure that the hips remain at a central position.

5.   **Knees:**

Stand tall, and try to bring the right knee all the way up to the chest. Now bring it down and try to touch your hip with your foot. Repeat this with the other leg. It is necessary to be in control while you perform this, so take your time.

6.   **Ankles:**

Raise one foot off the floor, point it in the forward direction, and rotate it in both directions. Repeat this exercise while maintaining the pivotal point at the ankles of each foot.

Chapter # 3: Pulse Raising, Targeted Mobility and Final Pulse Raising

The **Pulse Raising** stage of this regimen engages large muscle groups in order to increase your heart rate and body temperature. It is performed with the help of simple exercises like walking, jogging, and cycling. For instance, you may walk in or outside your house for 3 – 6 minutes, gently turning it to a jog for 2 minutes if you want.

Targeted Mobility on the other hand, are exercises that are focused on the part of the body that will be most engaged in the exercises, like the legs, when you're going to be running or the arms for swimming, etc. These exercises have similar range, as well as direction of rotation, as the exercise involved. The specific mobility exercise is dependent on the exercise and will therefore accompany the instructional manual of the exercise you are trying to do.

The **Final Pulse Raiser** will raise the heart rate and body temperature, further injecting a high-paced activity. For runners, the best pulse raiser would be to jog at a gradual pace to get the leg muscles ready for a high intensity run. For kick-boxers, it is best to perform fighting moves on a sand bag. For swimmers, a slow-paced swim would suffice and so on.

Next, perform the exercise and get ready to cool down.

Chapter # 4: Cooling Down

At the end of each session, it is vital to not come to a sudden stop. Once the session expires, slow your body down gradually using cool down techniques, followed by stretches. The purpose of a cool down is to return your body to the state from which it started. Contrary to a cool down session, if you abruptly stop the exercise, your heart would still pump blood at a higher rate, but the absence of a physical activity will result in the blood pooling in the limbs, and that will only cause dizziness. Stopping too slowly also causes sluggishness in the removal of waste products from the body, and that will hamper the recovery process and increase the likelihood of sore muscles the next morning. To prevent all this, you must perform a cool down exercise for just 5 minutes to allow the heart rate to return to normal. Cool down exercises include stretching, which are perfect to perform at high body temperatures. Something you would have achieved already due to the physical activity.

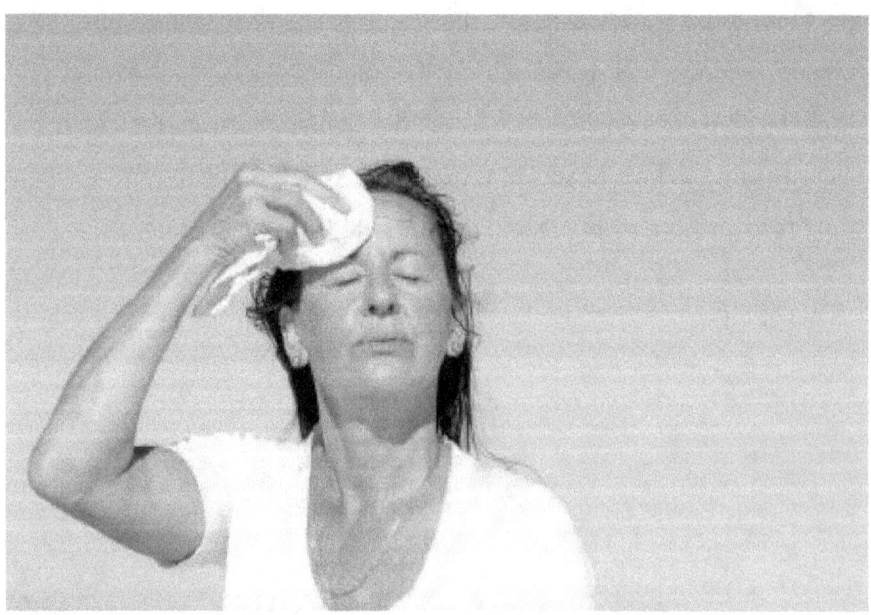

Good flexibility is a result of the perfect length in the muscles and the tissues surrounding the joint. Moreover, stretching is necessary to help the muscles relax, which would in turn help them to come back to the starting length. It has been found that muscles actually return to a contracted length if not cooled down properly, which can reduce their mobility. However, it must be noted that a brief cool down stretch would not improve the flexibility of muscles, and would only keep it at a constant level.

The following are ways that must be considered for a correct stretching session:

i.   Only stretch those muscles that have been warmed up thoroughly.

ii.   Breathe freely and always focus on being relaxed.

iii.   Slowly lengthen the muscle towards the point where you would start feeling pain. Give up at the point where a sensation of discomfort takes over and not pain.

iv.   Make sure you have correct body alignment and be aware of the muscle or the group of muscles you are focusing on when stretching.

v.   Avoid jerking or bouncing the joints and keep the movements as much in control as possible.

vi.   Hold the stretch position for 10 seconds; you must notice a relaxation or "give" feeling while performing it. If you do, hold the position for an extra 10 seconds.

vii.   Repeat each stretch exercise at least twice.

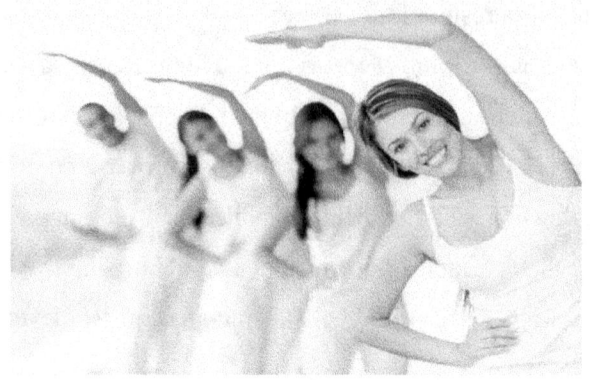

Chapter # 5: Upper Body Stretches

1. Neck:

Stand tall and use one of your hands to bend your head to the same side with focus being on the neck stretching out. To increase the stretch, make use of the hand to further pull the head.

2. Back & Shoulders:

Stand hip width apart and slightly bend your knees. Give your back a C shape by pushing away from the shoulders and the upper back providing a curve to it.

3. Chest:

Clasp your hands and position them behind your back. Pull your arms away from the back while keeping it as straight as possible with your shoulders down.

4. Shoulders:

Stand with the feet hip width apart, take your right arm from across the body, and use the crook of the left arm to grasp the right arm. Pull it towards your chest, gently, while making sure that the shoulders don't hunch up.

To give optimum stretch to the front and middle part of the shoulders, position yourself on all fours, sitting back on the haunches and extend your arms as far as possible.

5. Forearms:

Extend both the arms in front of the chest and use the right hand to press the fingers of the left hand backwards. Repeat the press part of the exercise first on the left hand and then on the right.

6.   **Triceps:**

Extend the right arm above the head, bending the elbow by dropping the forearm behind the head. Gently, apply force on the elbow with the left hand, backwards. Repeat with the other elbow.

7.   **Side Stretches:**

Stand hip distance apart focusing on the hips as the pivot, and take your torso towards one side, while sliding your hand along the thigh. If you wish to increase the amount of stretch, you may try bringing the free arm to the backside of your ear.

8.   **Lower back:**

Lie on the floor while bringing your knees towards your chest as if you are trying to contract yourself. Grab a hold of the shins and push yourself inwards initiating the stretch.

9.   **Modified Cobra:**

Lie chest down on the floor and rest your forearms on the floor with the elbow at a 90-degree angle to the forearms. Press your hipbone into the floor, allowing your back to ease in, then look forward and press your hipbone alternately into the ground.

Chapter # 6: Lower Body Stretches

1. **Quadriceps:**

    Stand tall and grab your right foot using your right hand, and try to take the foot behind you as far back as possible, so that it touches your hips. Keep your legs aligned and make sure that your back doesn't arch as you press the foot towards yourself.

2. **Calf:**

    Take a step worth 1 meter forward with the left leg whilst keeping the right one straight. Bend the knee which has landed 1 meter apart and press the hips forward, while keeping the right heel grounded. Ensure that the toes of the right foot point forward and not sideways. Bring the back leg closer to the front one and bend both knees so that the lower part of the back calf can stretch. Repeat this with the alternate setup.

3. **Hip Flexors:**

    Assume lunge position and press your back knee to the floor with the laces of your shoes facing downwards as well. Make sure that the torso is upright and lean into the font leg until there is a certain stretch feeling along the front line of the hip. To avoid extensive stress on the joint, make sure that the front knee does not go beyond the ankle. Repeat by swapping sides.

4. **Hamstrings:**

Stand tall with one leg extended outwards in front of you, with the foot resting on the ground. Keep the other knee bent and make sure that the hands are resting on this leg's thigh. Keep the abdominal part of the body gently contracted; repeat with the other side.

5.   **Hips:**

Bend your knees, raise your feet, and lie on your back. Put your left foot over your right thigh and connect your hands behind the right thigh so as to pull the legs towards the torso, stretching out the right hip. Repeat while swapping sides.

6.   **Groin:**

While sitting on the floor, bring the feet together so that both the soles touch each other. Press down on the thighs using your elbows and then extend your legs out sideways, as far as possible, to a point where you're comfortable. Keep your back straight and try to reach the toe of each leg using your hands by pressing your body one way and then the other.

It must be noted that research has shown no significant benefit to the body as a result of stretches before warm ups. In fact, dynamic methods like dedicated stretch routines are much more effective at preparing the body. Still, if you must exercise before stretching, don't press a muscle for more than 5 seconds as it can actually switch off the muscle, and inhibit performance greatly. It is for this reason that the army exercises now include dedicated stretch days to improve a soldier's performance. Therefore, if you can put some time aside to stretch, you can only benefit.

Targeted Warm ups

The following chapters will contain warm up exercises that will reflect a particular physical activity, and should be carried out only by their respective athletes. The types of physical activities covered are:

1.   Low Impact Exercises,

2.   Aerobic Exercises,

3.   Cardio-Kickboxing Exercises,

Chapter # 1: Low Impact Exercises

1.   **Overhead Raise with Pec Fly:**

With the elbows bent to an angle of 90 degrees, raise each elbow up to shoulder level and then move them back in a way that they align with the body. The arms should now look like a field goal post. This is the starting position, after which, try to bring your elbows together as if you were about to execute a pec fly. Once your elbows touch each other, gently lift both the arms over your head. Reverse the exercise to get back where you're starting.

2.   **Chest Press:**

Imagine that you are performing a push-up in space, right in front of the body. Once you achieve the starting position, proceed with an overhead shoulder press, making sure that a narrow hand stance is used all the way. Keep the elbows tucked in during the press so that the triceps are engaged.

3.   **Calf Raise:**

Execute a standing calf raise while rotating your head so that it looks over the right shoulder. Perform 10 reps to the right, switch positions, and then perform 10 reps to the left. This exercise is done to warm up the calves and simultaneously provides a good amount of motion to the neck. However, do NOT turn your neck in an alternating manner, as this will only cause dizziness.

4.   **Toe Tap to the Front:**

Stand at shoulder width, gradually lifting your right knee and rotating the hip so that it can touch the inside of the right foot using the left hand. Repeat this with the other side by touching the right hand on the inside of the right foot. Repeat 8 - 10 times.

5.   **Line-pulling to the front:**

Stand slightly greater than shoulder width and perform a partial squat. The squat part is necessary if you want to successfully target your legs during the warm up. Now, simulate as if you were pulling a line from a ship (tug-of-war). Change positions from right to left, etc.

Chapter # 2: Basic Aerobic Exercises

1.   **Basic March & Wide March:**

Perform a four-count march with a normal stance and afterwards widen up your stance. Now, perform a widened four-count march. Repeat 4 – 5 times.

2.   **Box Step:**

Assume normal stance. Now step forward and out using the right foot, then forward and out using the left one. Bring your left foot back to the starting position and then bring the right foot back to the initial point. The overall movement that you make must be that of a V. Perform this exercise similar to a 4 count.

3.   **Toe Tap with Overhead Reach:**

Tap the feet sideways. Take your arm to the right and then perform an overhead reach to the left. Now take the left arm and perform an overhead reach to the right. Repeat this entire sequence with a 4-count call for 5-7 repetitions.

4.   **Grape Wine:**

Assume normal stance and step to the right by crossing the left foot behind the right one. Move the right foot a step to the right in order to assume normal stance and finish it up by tapping the left foot next to the right. Perform the same sequence, but to the left using a four count call.

5.   **Squat with Kick:**

Carrying out your arms in a guarded position, first perform a squat and then a left front kick, followed by another squat and then a right kick. This will improve balance in your body.

Chapter # 3: Cardio-Kickboxing Exercises

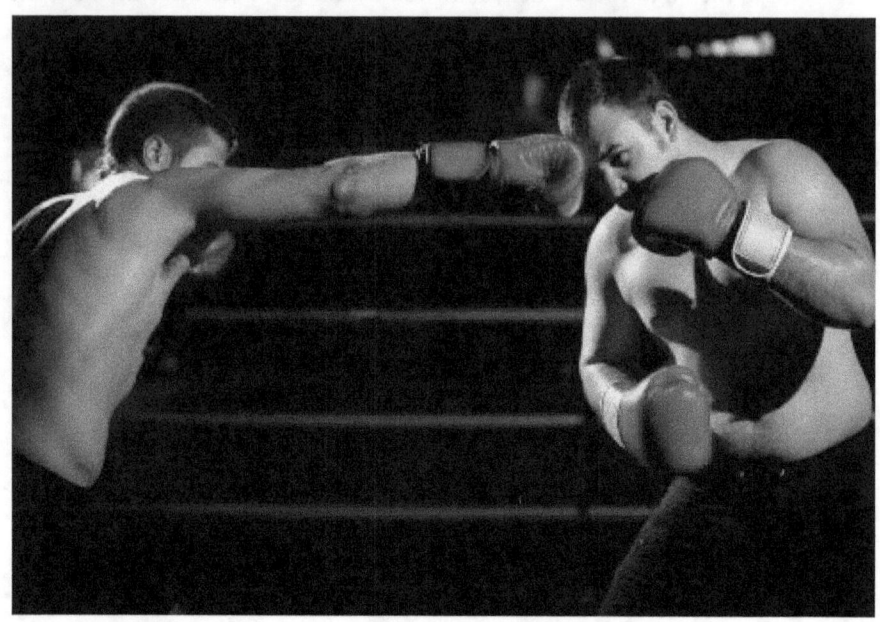

1. **Speed Bag:**

    Clinch your fists, raise your elbows up to the shoulders, and act as if you were punching a bag right in front of you. Make sure to rotate your fists in the process. After performing this at shoulder level, set the new level above your heat. As the temperature of the body rises, you may perform a boxer's shuffle to increase the intensity of the exercise.

2. **Straight Jab:**

    Standing with the left hip forward, bring both fists in front of your face in a well-guarded position. Now, take your left hand and perform a quick jab right at the front, and return to the initial position. You may perform a boxer's shuffle to increase the intensity of the exercise. The purpose of this warm up exercise is to get the upper body warm, especially the biceps, shoulders, and triceps.

3. **Straight Jab-Side Jab:**

With the left hip facing forward, take the left fist and throw a jab to the front. Then use the right foot as a pivot and jab to the side. Pivot once again to return to the starting point. Repeat 5 – 6 times.

4. **Alternating hooks:**

Stand a little wider than shoulder width with your hands in a guarded stance, and start tapping your feet, sideways. Once sufficient rhythm is obtained, throw a hook to the left as you tap the left foot, and then do the same with the right foot. Remember to have a pivotal position at the back foot so that the knee does not have to absorb extra strain. A hook is basically a bent punch, and it is initiated with the arms in the guarded stance. With the right arm bent, bring the elbow backwards and rotate the shoulder so that the fist is positioned right at the midline of the body; the forearm should be shoulder level and parallel to the deck.

5. **Upper Cut:**

Position the feet at a slightly wider length than the shoulders and begin to tap your feet sideways. Once rhythm is obtained, throw a left upper cut as soon as the left foot is tapped and a right upper cut when the right foot is tapped. This is one of the basics of cardio-kickboxing exercise.

Conclusion

Warm ups are essential for an injury free workout: that was the topic of this book and that has been proven right. Warming up is a core phase of any exercise or physical activity, as it can start to bring the body into the required form. As a person proceeds with his/her warm up, the body starts to loosen up, the blood flow increases, and the muscles get ready for a high intensity session. In addition to warming up, the book also tells about the added benefit of stretching to the body and the problems surrounding it. The book illustrates both warming up and stretching exercises so a person with additional interest for his/her muscles can benefit more. Moreover, targeted warm up exercises for different physical activities have also been given to ensure proper and thorough understanding.

Stay safe, best of Luck!

References

http://fotolia.com/id/39676947

http://fotolia.com/id/46908327

http://fotolia.com/id/45156048

http://nl.123rf.com/photo_14580629_groep-mensen-opwarmen-in-de-sportschool.html?term=warming%20up%20exercises

http://nl.123rf.com/photo_20105565_groep-van-mensen-die-het-beoefenen-van-yoga-en-lachend.html?term=stretching

http://nl.123rf.com/photo_16766152_portret-van-gestresst-en-uitgeput-zoekt-vrouw-van-middelbare-leeftijd-probeert-om-het-gezicht-af-te-.html?term=cool%20down%20exercise

http://nl.123rf.com/photo_21825362_boxer-met-behulp-van-enkele-jabs-om-zijn-tegenstander-te-slaan-en-win-de-doos-wedstrijd.html?term=boxing

Author Bio

Muhammad Usman is a distinguished medical graduate of Allama Iqbal medical college (AIMC). He is a professional writer who has been in the field for more than 4 years. During this time he has produced 10,000+ articles, blogs and eBooks on various niches related to diseases, health, fitness, nutrition and well-being. He is a regular contributor to several journals related to medicine and surgery. He is the editor of several journals and newspapers.

Check out some of the other JD-Biz Publishing books

Gardening Series on Amazon

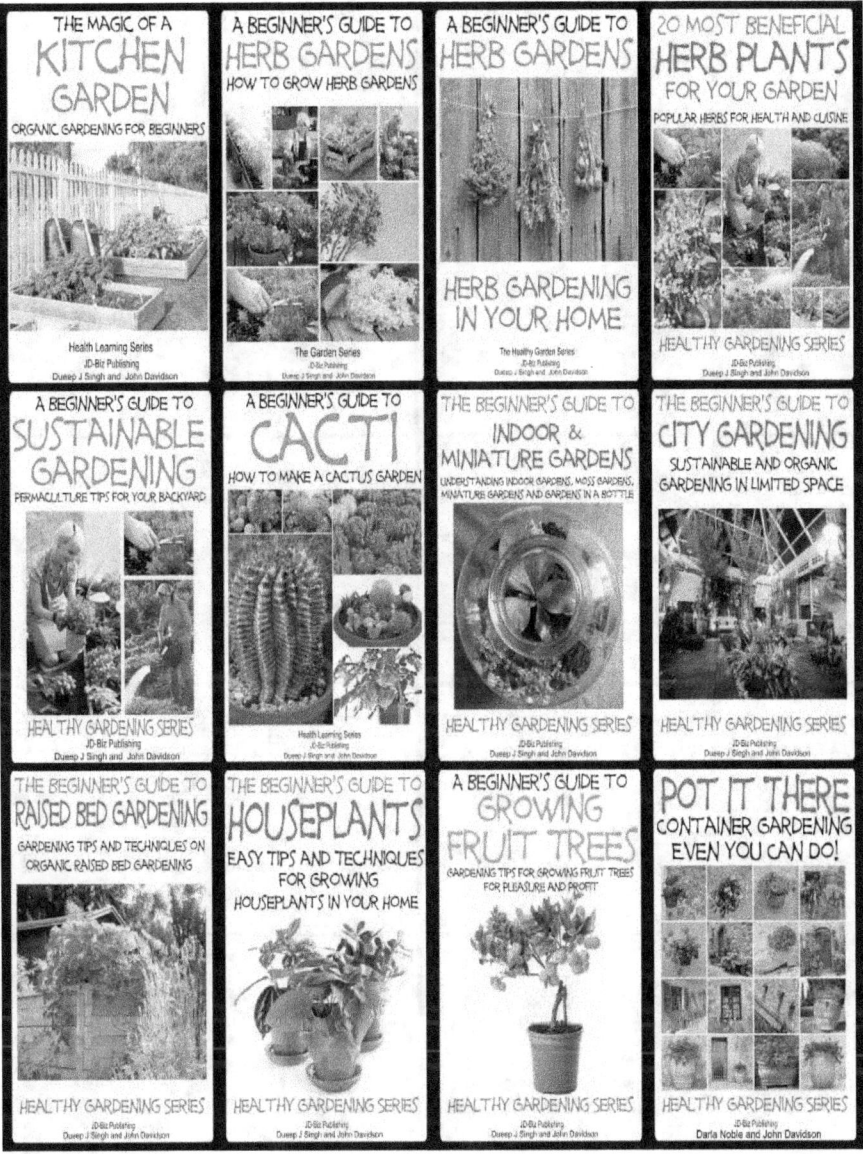

Health Learning Series

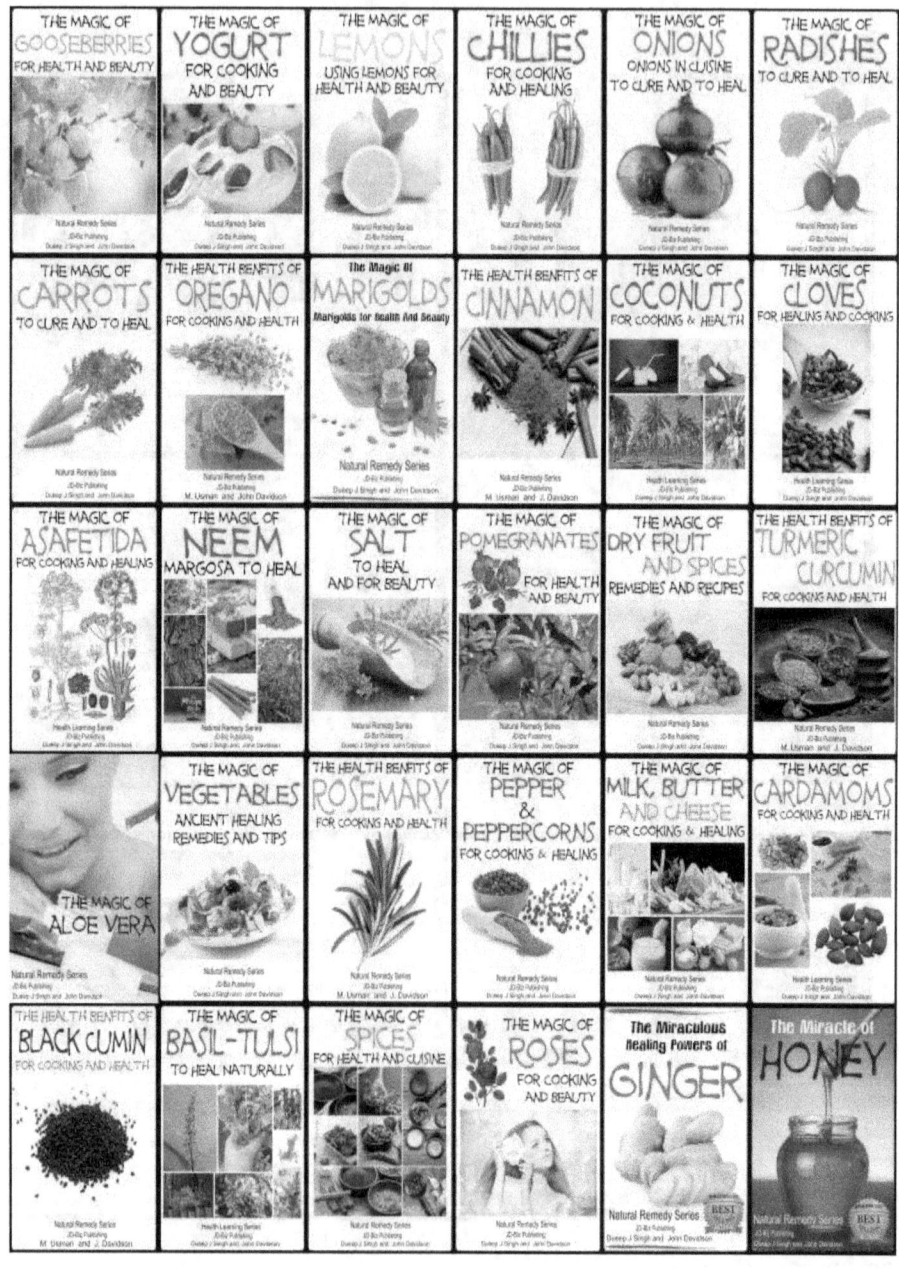

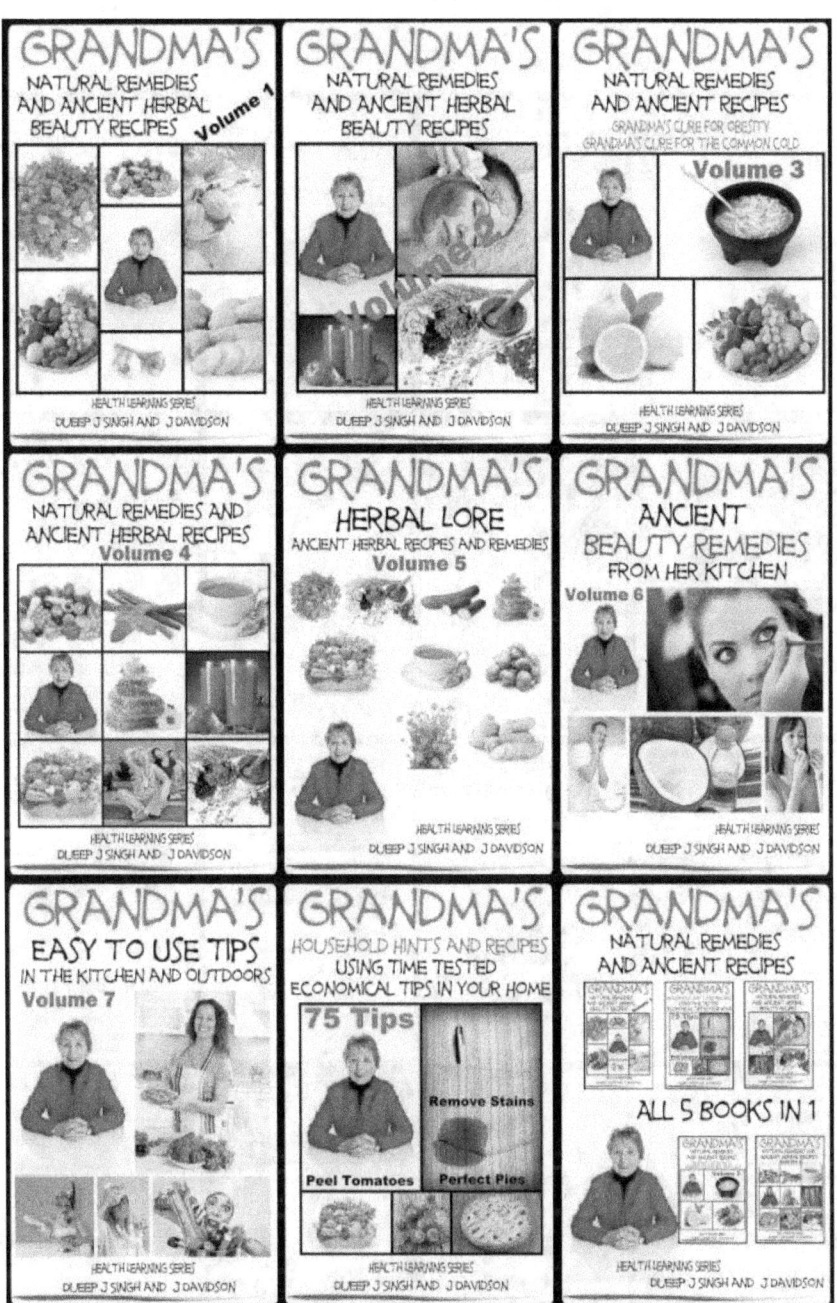

Country Life Books

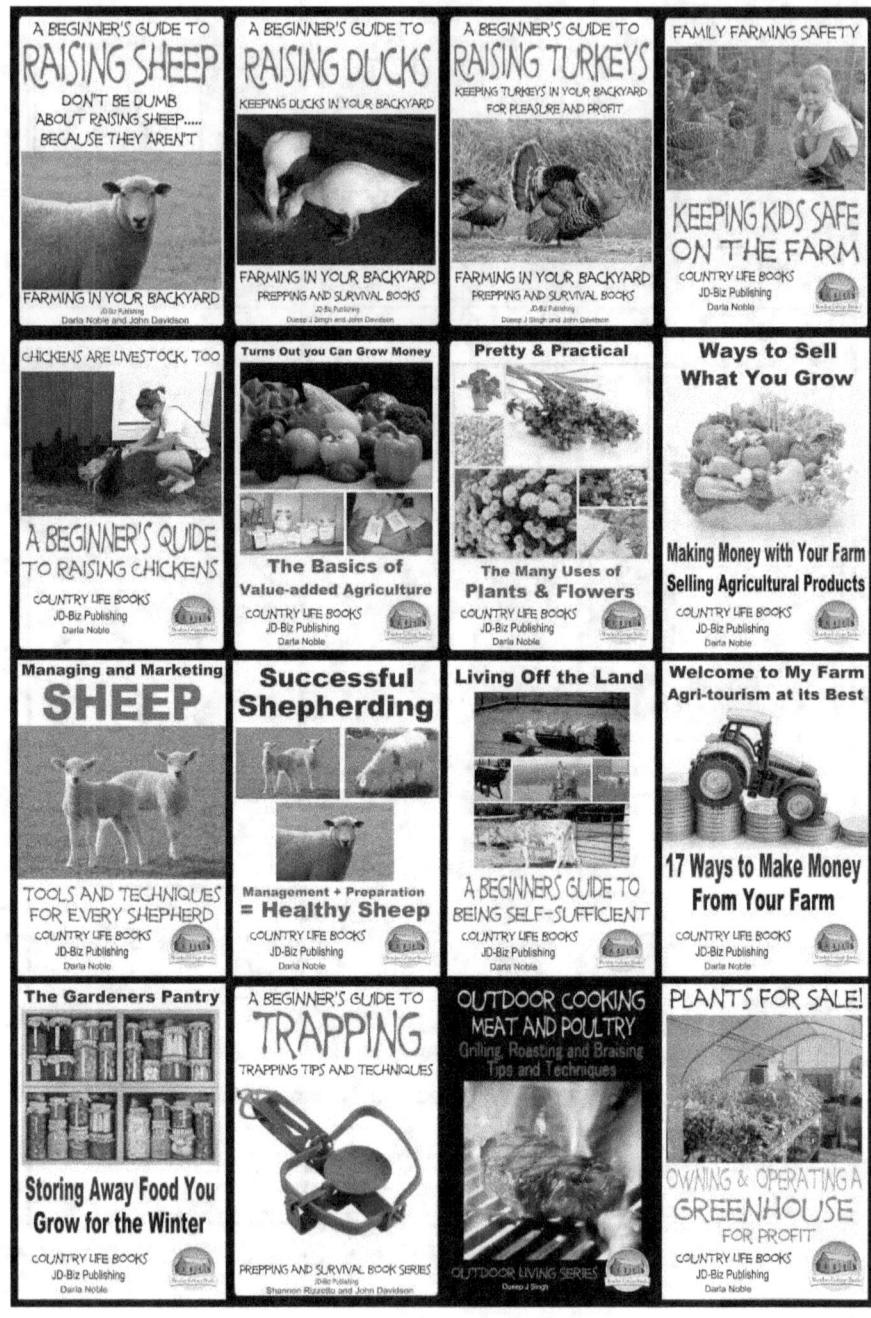

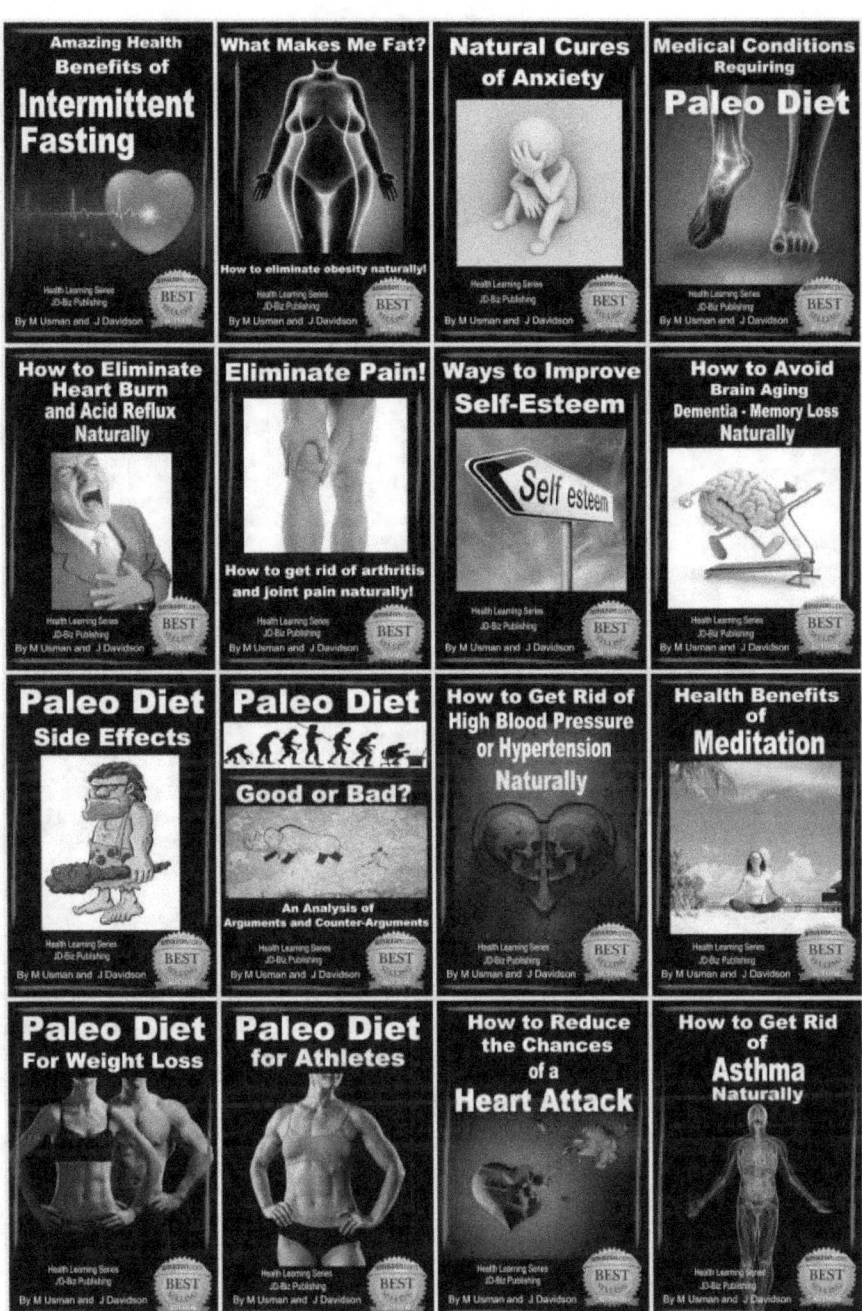

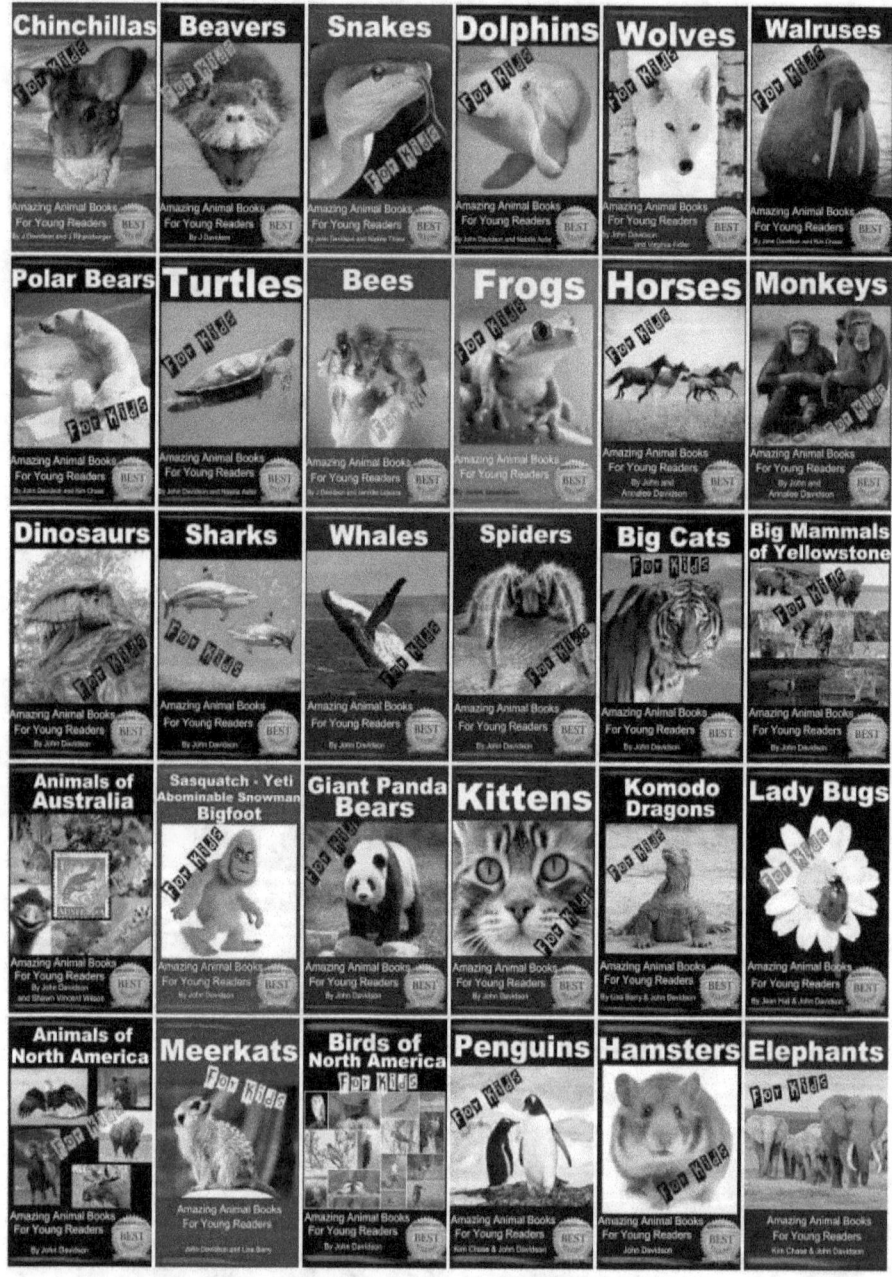

Learn To Draw Series

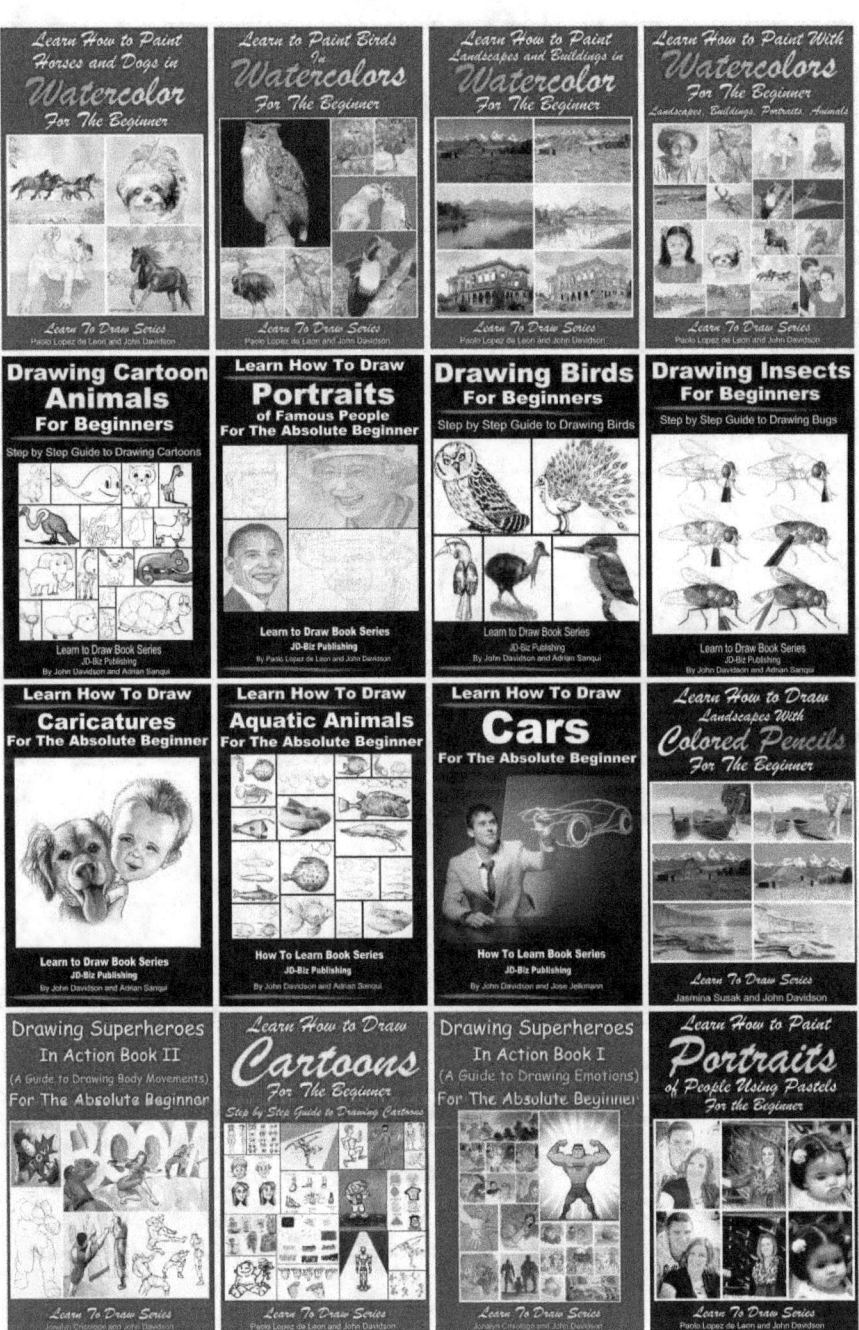

How to Build and Plan Books

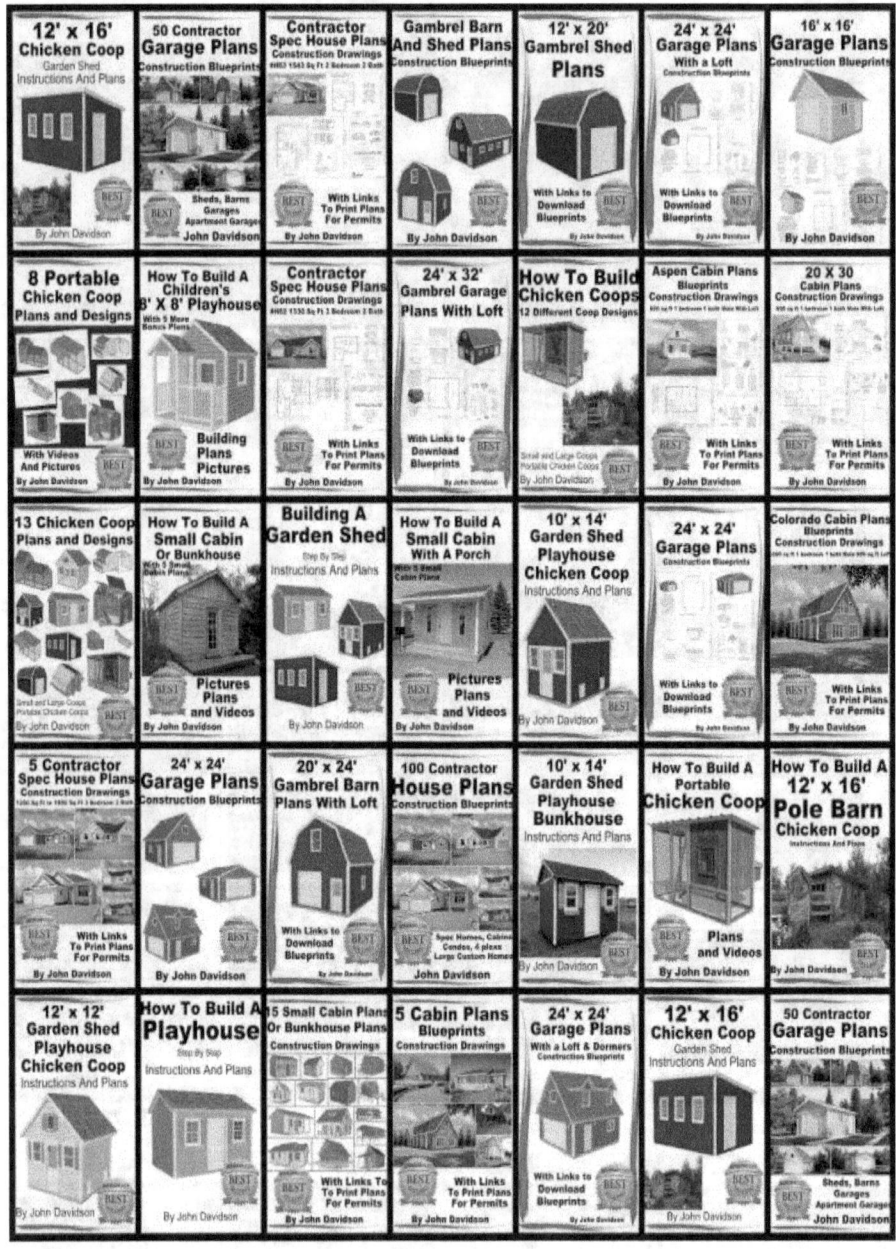

Entrepreneur Book Series

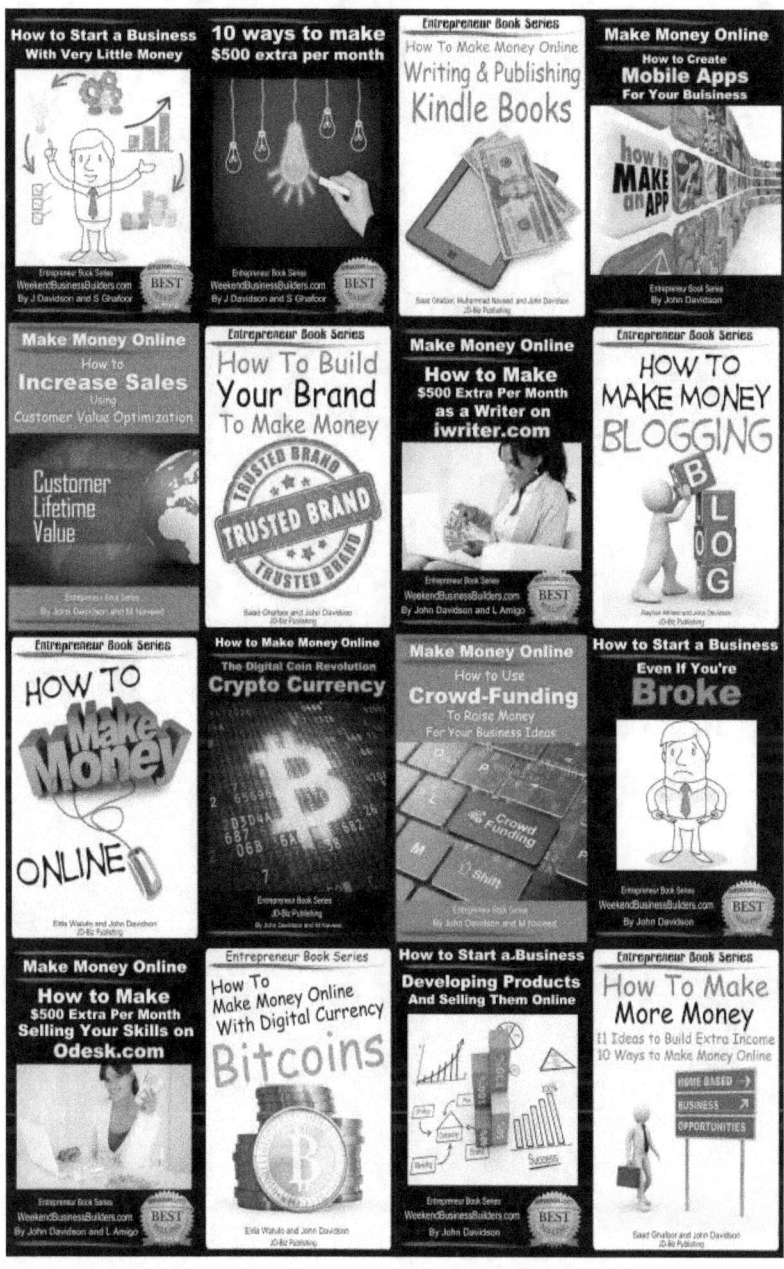

Our books are available at

1. Amazon.com

2. Barnes and Noble

3. Itunes

4. Kobo

5. Smashwords

6. Google Play Books

Publisher

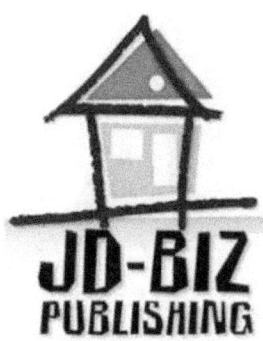

JD-Biz Corp

P O Box 374

Mendon, Utah 84325

http://www.jd-biz.com/

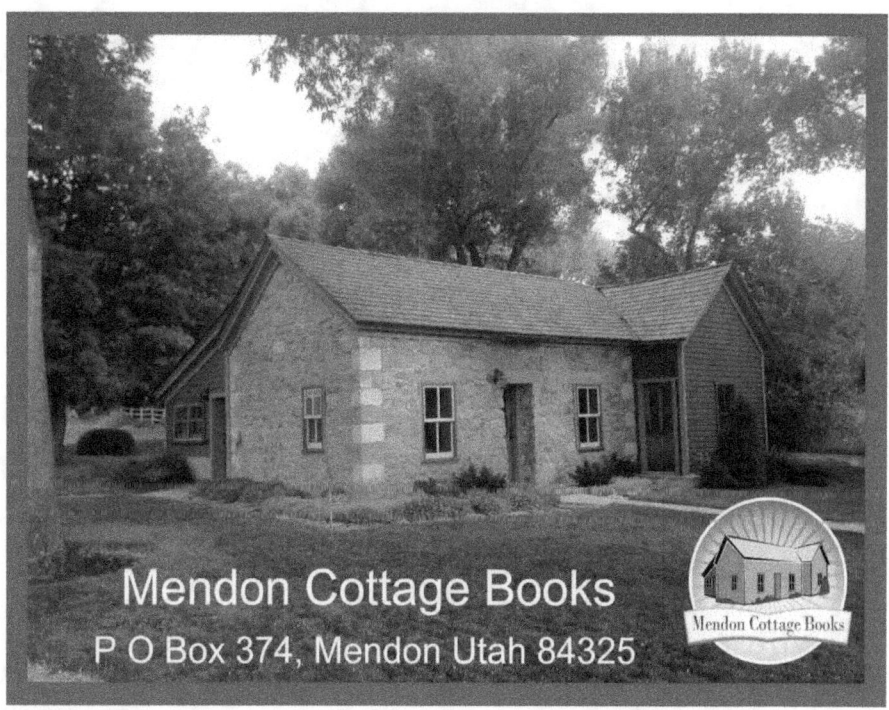

Mendon Cottage Books

P O Box 374, Mendon Utah 84325

Mendon Cottage Books

www.ingramcontent.com/pod-product-compliance
Lightning Source LLC
Chambersburg PA
CBHW070508290526
45790CB00003B/1145